Simply

GW00857542

by Sofia Bothwell

Simply Full © Sofia Bothwell 2012

Disclaimer: The information in this book is a form of sharing my own direct experience and is for information purposes only and certainly not given as a substitute for qualified medical advice.

INTRODUCTION

Being slim is possible. Being slim is a reality I've enjoyed for over twenty years. Being free from compulsive eating, being free from the obsession with size, shape and food is something I want everyone who has ever struggled with their weight to experience. May this book help you and guide you, bring you the tools, ideas and ways of relating to yourself and food that will enable, within you, that profound transformation that I experienced a long time ago - a transformation that I can see is possible for all of you – the transformation into your permanently slim self.

Wishing you many blessings as you get slimmer and stay slim for good.

Much love, Sofia

For further information on Sofia's work contact:

Sofia2227@gmail.com

www.sofiabothwell.co.uk

☯

Where to begin? We begin with the hunger and fullness sensations, becoming familiar with them, and abiding by them. This is our task now. Over the next few weeks and months you will be following the guidance of your hunger and fullness sensations.

You will also be getting more in tune with your emotions. All methods of weight loss that try to cut out the *eating when full* without dealing with the underlying emotional issues, are doomed to failure. So let's take the route of success. I would like you to ask yourself 'Am I ready to face up to, and resolve, the emotions that are behind my habit of eating when physically full?' I hope your answer is a resounding 'Yes!' For this affirmative answer will prepare you for the most essential part of losing excess weight for good! And I want total and utter success for you, just as I have experienced in my own life after years of struggling with an obsession with size, shape and dysfunctional eating patterns.

When I stopped dieting, and endeavored to stop eating when physically full, whilst being aware of the emotions I felt *as* I stopped when full, relief came, my excess pounds were shed, and a relaxed, happy, healthy relationship to food, my body, and eating, occurred. This is what I know every single one of you can experience - freedom from *food when full*.

So let's start! The most important question to ask yourself when you want to lose weight is – *Am I hungry?* Asking yourself - *Am I hungry?* - anytime you think about food or eating, is the best way to connect with the innate intelligence of your stomach. Your stomach is always relaying information to you about your food intake, and letting you know when enough is enough as far as consumption of food is concerned.

Following the innate intelligence of one's own stomach is what I teach, it's what got me slim and has kept me slim for over twenty years. If you eat when you have a fullness sensation obviously telling you that you are physically full, you will gain weight. It is as simple as that. Over and above the *type of food* you eat, it is *stopping when full* that will get you and keep you slim. It is through stopping when full that you are allowing your body to find and maintain its own natural weight.

Eating when *hungry* keeps us alive. Eating when _full_ on the other hand, is addiction to food, suppresses emotion, makes, and keeps us fat. Eating when *full* serves the purpose of suppressing life's uncomfortable emotions, and what is suppressed pops up again and again, in ever more annoying ways, for it is crying out to be felt, and resolved for good. Therefore, when we stop when full, we are no longer suppressing uncomfortable feelings and emotions, we are experiencing them instead. The next step is resolving – resolving those feelings and emotional issues that could drive us to the fridge when full. Once we are aware that we will be experiencing our previously suppressed uncomfortable emotions as we give up eating when full, we are not so perturbed when some uncomfortable emotions arise. We are so accustomed to thinking – *Ah everything will be brilliant as I start losing the weight! And I will feel great when slimmer,* we are really thrown when the reality of an intense, uncomfortable emotion or two, presents itself to us accompanying our slimmer body size. We think a slim body is supposed to go along with a fabulous life where all goes well and I feel good all the time. We think a slim body is not supposed to go along with a regular life and sometimes feeling lousy. We do not know what to do when this issue presents itself to us. We are convinced that it's not supposed to feel bad, it's not supposed to feel difficult, stressful or boring when you are slim – or is it? This is the myth I am exploring and replacing with the truth of the matter – *Stopping when full* allows us to get, and stay, slim, but *stopping when full* involves us feeling lousy emotionally sometimes. It is our task to navigate that lousiness! So, in being prepared for the road to slimness to sometimes be a bit of an emotionally bumpy ride, we can continue…

A lot of what I teach is common sense wisdom, remind yourself of the following common sense wisdom often, for it leads to good health:

Eating only when physically hungry allows healthy digestion. Eating only when physically hungry, nourishes the body efficiently. Eating only when physically hungry is good for the metabolism. Eating only when physically hungry is natural. Eating only when physically hungry is a wise choice. Eating only when physically hungry is essential for good energy levels. Eating only when physically hungry allows us to feel our emotions more easily, both pleasant and unpleasant ones, and feeling emotions is the hallmark of good health in many, many ways.

Stop when full, stop when full, stop when full! The only thing that prevents us stopping eating when physically full, is an emotion. An unresolved emotion. Feel the emotion, resolve the emotion, and you can stop eating when physically full more easily, because your focus is on the real issue – emotions, not food, not taste, not willpower, but emotion, emotion, emotion. Losing weight permanently, is indeed, very much about what goes on, in our hearts and minds, as much as it is about what goes into our mouths and stomachs.

Many people say to me - 'But isn't it just because the food tastes so good that I eat so much of it when full?' Well, food tastes even better when we are hungry *and fancy* that particular type of food. A little overindulgence, occasionally, like at Christmas or a celebration, an extra spoonful or two of a really delicious soup, or desert when full – yes – but any more than that, and you are eating for some sort of emotional reason. Look back on any time you ate until positively stuffed, and you will find the emotional cause. Ask yourself – How did I feel emotionally just prior to overeating? This way you have added insight into your eating patterns.

How am I going to resolve those emotions, so I no longer *eat when full* because of them? Well, anytime you feel like *eating when physically full*, ask yourself immediately - 'What feeling is this?' And then, once you have an idea of what feeling or emotion is there, ask yourself - 'Given the fact I feel this way, what would I like to do now?' This simple formula is quite literally your road map out of *eating when full,* and the region called 'excess weight' can be left behind for good. Thus you start to navigate the internal waters of consciousness, finding your way in life without the crutch of *eating when full* to suppress your unresolved emotional stuff.

Eating when *physically full* is food addiction. Eating when physically full suppresses feelings. Eating when physically full serves to numb us, or distract us, from our feelings. Eating when physically full causes excess weight. Eating when physically full can create indigestion, bloating, gas and nausea. No one can lose weight permanently if any eating when physically full is going on.

Eat when hungry, stop when full. Eat when hungry, stop when full. Let this be your new, much repeated mantra, your new habit, and your new modus operandi. Let the question - Am I physically hungry? - be your embedded automatic response to any thought of food or eating. So, when the thought occurs - *Oh I fancy a sandwich* - let your automatic reaction be: 'Am I physically hungry?' Likewise, for the thought – *Got to get some chips for tea* – respond with 'Am I physically hungry?' For it is through asking this question that we regain our direct link to our built-in, weight regulators – the hunger and fullness sensations.

Some people say to me – *But it seems like I am <u>denying</u> myself food when I try to stop eating when full.*

It is true we are *abstaining* from food when full, but in so doing we are giving ourselves the opportunity to gain freedom from the specific eating that causes excess weight. I ask them to consider the word *deny* in this context to be an inaccurate term. Rather we are giving ourselves *freedom from* food when full. We are also gaining an understanding of why we would even want to *eat when full* in the first place. Eating when full is dysfunctional eating and an eating disorder – we are healing that eating disorder by gaining the ability to stop eating when full. This is freedom, not denial. And when we are physically <u>hungry</u> we have the full range of foods and beverages to choose from.

Emotional issues are part of life, and if we eat when full because of them, we not only gain weight, we also deny ourselves a bit of life. We numb ourselves to that chunk of our life experience. Life does not like to be numbed, denied or shoved into suppression, so it becomes, ultimately, an unpleasant experience. Unpleasant due to the excess weight we carry, the tummy ache we may experience, not to mention the excess gas, or pain of indigestion, all because we ate when full because of emotional issues instead of facing up to and resolving those emotional issues.

I am sure you have often heard or even used the phrase - *Biscuits are my downfall.* Or - *Chocolate is my downfall.* Well, as all-powerful as biscuits and chocolate can be, they do not have the power, in and of themselves, to cause anyone's downfall. What does? Our inability, through no fault of our own, to recognise, feel and resolve the emotional stuff that drives us to eat when full. Biscuits, even chocolate ones, do not have the power to make us overindulge in them. But it is true, we are rendered helpless to resist a binge on biscuits when we *know of no other way of coping* other than overindulgence. Throughout this book are the ideas, tips and tools to give you access to many other *means of coping* so that you have alternatives to the overindulgence, and you *can* gain freedom from eating when full.

Chocolate isn't a sweet, it is a medicine, just ask any premenstrual female and she will tell you – That chocolate bar in her hand, its use is medicinal. Well joking aside, there is some truth in this. Dr Christiane Northrup (author of Women's Bodies Women's Wisdom and The Wisdom of Menopause) states that when we are premenstrual it is like the tide being out, and we see all our emotional shipwrecks. The trick is to wisely use this premenstrual time to clean up our emotional shipwrecks not turn away from them by eating when full, but a little bit of chocolate when hungry is okay – for medicinal purposes.

There is an old Buddhist saying - Feelings are like clouds in the sky, they pass. Our job is to *feel those feelings as they pass through us*, this leads us not only to permanent slimness but also gives us good physical health, emotional well being, and a stronger sense of self. To help with this *processing,* or *feeling* of feelings, spend a day being extra aware of how you feel. Jot down, in a small notebook or phone the feelings you become aware of as you go about your daily routine. This could be annoyance at a co-worker, or joy at a child's smile. Just spend as much time as you can, being aware of how you feel emotionally.

What do you think would be different if you were slim? Make a list, or just consider it for a moment. Now, what do you need to do, what perspective do you need to take, in order for *that difference,* to be in your life now, regardless of your size and shape? Really ponder this, for it is vitally important in the process of allowing / achieving true and lasting slimness. So, make a list of the very real differences, that *you* feel, being slim, will bring in its wake. List all the positive associations that being slim conjures up for you, and then list what it takes to bring 'em in now!

For example: Being slim will mean I am more attractive. How can I bring that 'attractiveness' into my life now? Well, people like my smile so I could smile more often. I could take more time with my hair and wear a little lipstick now and then. These are simple steps, and simple steps are easy to make.

Feelings are energy and energy cannot be destroyed, it changes, but it cannot be destroyed.

For example: The feeling of anger, when felt, and <u>not</u> dumped on someone by yelling at them, can turn into purposefulness. So, as our anger dissipates, we find we have the ability to take action, to heal the thing we are angry about, some injustice has been done, some need is not being met when we feel angry. Pinpoint the need and seek to meet the need, and the feeling of purposefulness is born within you from <u>not</u> suppressing or dumping your anger, but simply being aware of it, willing to feel it and process it healthily. In private, beating the mattress with your fists or doing a silent scream; going for a brisk walk or run, can all help you healthily process the powerful, and sometimes frightening, feeling of anger. Removing yourself from the person or situation that is causing you to feel anger is often helpful too, and far more effective than yelling and screaming at them, slamming doors or slamming your hands down on the table in a dramatic gesture - these are all ways of dumping anger, and are abusive to those in the room with you, thus not conducive to healthy relationships or friendships. In fact, I would always distance myself from anyone who regularly behaves in such a way.

A slim figure is just that - a slim figure, a body size that is the result of our food intake. Now, we certainly have associated it with a load of other stuff, like confidence, beauty, grace, attractiveness, the ability to pull, desirability, success and energy; even a good life, things going well and having-it-all, have been associated with the ever elusive slim figure. But the truth is: A slim figure, is just that – a slim figure, the plain and simple result of our food intake, and no guarantee of that load of aforementioned positive stuff.

In fact a slim figure, in and of itself, rarely delivers confidence, attractiveness, success, or feeling good about oneself. If we do not already possess those qualities at our bigger size, they cannot magically appear when we are slim just by virtue of that slimness. Or, if it does deliver them, it is on a superficial level, and often short-lived. The emotional journey from a *lack of these qualities* to *an abundance of these qualities,* has to be taken in order to make them permanent qualities within ourselves whatever our size and shape.

Do not wait for slimness to do it for you, because the truth is – it can't. Do what for you? Give you all those things that you believe will happen when you are slim. Take a moment and list them. Many believe that once they are slim the perfect relationship will come along, or vast improvement will enter their present marriage. The unconscious and often conscious presumption that *relationships will be better when I'm slim* is a myth we all have to deal with as we endeavor to lose our excess weight for good. Slimness alone - does not make relationships or anything else better - resolving emotional issues does. For example: You could be slim and have chronic fatigue syndrome, or receive a diagnosis of breast cancer – this can happen and are examples of being slim and all not going very well. Extreme financial problems, or a lover leaving does indeed happen to the slim attractive woman. So know that 'slimness' is not the answer to your problems - it is a body size. Slimness is not the answer to your problems - resolving emotional issues, is!

Addiction has been described, as *the inability to act on one's own behalf,* in other words, not being able to act on the healthy choice that we know is available. Why would we choose an unhealthy choice, such as eating when full, when the healthy choice (to simply stop when full) is seemingly, readily available? Well, we are out of control. The healthy choice *is* impossible to make, the craving to eat when full *is* so strong that the compulsive eater cannot stop eating even if she wants to. Not beating yourself up over sometimes being out of control around food is part of changing this. Another part of changing our *inability to stop when full* is to know, that what drives us to eat when full is the unconscious (sometimes conscious) urge, to suppress our emotions. It is like two urges are going on at once. (1) The urge (compulsion) to numb emotion and eat when full. And (2) The urge (desire) to stop eating, but risk feeling uncomfortable emotionally.

When we stop when full without actively addressing the emotional issues, or at least being prepared to feel difficult emotions associated with some problem or dilemma in our life, then we are left high and dry with these difficult emotions. Ease comes directly through pinpointing and resolving the emotional issue. We can start by asking ourselves - *What emotion is this, and given the fact I feel this way, what would I like to do now?*

So, even if it usually feels like you have little or no control over your *habit of eating when full*, just bear in mind, that on some level, it is indeed a choice, and that you are in the process of learning how to make another choice. What we are doing, in learning how to lose weight this way, is learning how to regain control over when we stop eating. We do this by asking - 'What feeling is this?' when we have the urge to eat when full. This question acts like a knife cutting the cords that would pull us into eating when full. This question immediately disperses the fog of the semi-conscious, automatic, dysfunctional behavior of eating when full. Again ask yourself: 'What feeling is this?' Even as you are spooning into your mouth, food you know, you are eating when already full. Persist with the question: 'What feeling is this?' It is through repeatedly practicing this, that you can be more in tune with the specific emotions that drive you to eat when full, and develop the ability to stop when full as you actively consider other ways to deal with these emotions.

So cease any self-condemnation for being out of control. That very phrase 'out of control' has very negative connotations. It is more conducive to changing dysfunctional eating habits, to view eating when full, as simply a choice we made when we felt we had no choice. Once our skill at being able to handle our emotions increases, the urge, and even uncontrollable compulsion to *eat when full* because of them, diminishes. This, to me, is a dissolving of withdrawal symptoms. Many people think that withdrawal symptoms simply cannot be avoided and only in time they fade away, or we learn to bear them with extreme discomfort; however in my own experience when I have learned to handle my emotions in healthier ways, the cravings and withdrawal symptoms either greatly reduce or disappear altogether.

Alternative means of coping. In my own journey I have sought out and practiced many healthy, *alternative means of coping*. Rebirthing, a form of breathwork has been a big healer in my life. 'The Work' of Byron Katie, Bach Flower Remedies, Sound Healing, Affirmations of Louise Hay, books on Positive Thinking. All of which I throw your way as suggested tools to see if they resonate with you. I also encourage you to seek out your own, healthy, *alternative means of coping*. They will come in the form of *that which you are interested in*, fascinated about and are drawn towards. So discovering, paying attention to, and involving yourself in what interests you is not frivolous, but essential to living a contented, healthy and fulfilled life. We do not tend to overindulge in anything when we are basically at ease with life, on top of our emotional stuff, and involved in pursuits that interest us as much as time, resources, bank balance and improvisation allow.

I cannot stress enough the importance of doing what you love as a necessary part of what combines together to create a life free from eating when full and being overweight. Being involved in what you love, to me, *is* creativity. Often we feel we do not have the time to be creative, or we feel we have too many outside pressures from work, or family, to adequately devote time and finances to what we love. So, if challenging times occur, or are the norm, I've discovered that just knowing that *it can all go in my favor* is a great belief system to operate from, for we truly are like computers, running a program. Our thoughts and what we believe to be true about ourselves, really is the program that runs our life over and above outside circumstances.

Just the other day I watched a pair of beautiful large buzzards with such a large wingspan that they sailed majestically where smaller birds flap frantically or cannot even reach. The thought came to me – *Look! It is the same air current, it is the same sky in which* *all birds fly, but these two, with such grace and beauty soar like they are lord and lady over all that is below. It is your positive, follow-your-heart perspective that gives you your huge wings to ride the air currents of life with grace, whereas negative, fear-filled perspectives shrink your wing size, creating difficulty and effort.*

I further thought – *These majestic birds are supported by all that is around them, the land... the trees.* So too in life, all that is around *you* can support you. Look at what you have and where you want to go. The circumstances can grow into part of the journey that gets you there. Through a change in your perspective, a change in the thoughts you are believing about a situation, person or place you become a blessing to yourself and that situation, person or place just by your attitude and presence there. You can leave difficult situations and difficult people if you need to. You can, once you are coming from a place of integrity (not domination or bullying, nor being a victim) more easily glean what you desire from that situation, person or place. Solutions appear that are of benefit to all concerned, and win / win situations become the norm in your life, and in the lives of those around you. Not without its challenges, but you again, will rise above those challenges, use those challenges (or something within the challenge) to your advantage in some way. Through increased awareness of your situation you are more easily able to leave anything, anyone, or any habit behind. An inner strength is already there to make any change you need to make, to follow your very own heart-felt desires. The bottom line is, if you are in an abusive situation - leave!

Creativity – What is creativity? It's to be engaged in that which brings you joy. To ask yourself – What would I like to do now? – is to invite creativity into your life in a very real way, and it is a partner in healing the habit of eating when full. The other partner in healing the habit of eating when physically full of food, is - feeling feelings. This, in no uncertain terms, is the road to true and lasting slimness.

Intuition replaces cravings as our *prompting into action* mechanism, that we trust, and follow. Our cravings tell us to eat when full, drink alcohol or smoke. Our intuition can guide us to the healthy alternatives. This is the shift we are making as we give up eating when full. Consider this - it is the *craving* to eat when full, that is the unhealthy prompt, to the unhealthy action of eating when full. So, now we are endeavoring to ignore *that* prompt as the unwise choice that it is, while we gain practice in tuning into the healthy *prompt into action,* by asking ourselves the aforementioned questions: What feeling is this? And Given the fact I feel this way what would I like to do now? And we can do this at any time, not just when we feel the craving to eat when physically full.

I remember in my early twenties, I could literally feel the pain of heartbreak in my chest when a cherished relationship was falling apart. My way of coping was no longer eating when full, but unfortunately I, for two years, took up smoking again in order to numb the pain, but all the while I asked myself: How can I resolve this?

We ask the question, life gives us the answer. I felt strongly that I had to leave my then boyfriend, and, eventually I did.

Then one day a friend handed me the book 'Women Who Love Too Much' by Robin Norwood. This book showed me how addiction occurs in relationships. The other person, wishing and hoping they will change, becomes your addiction. Like all addictions it serves the purpose of being a huge distraction from our own unresolved issues. So in coming back to addressing my own unresolved issues, some of them old, half-forgotten, hurts and wounds, and using Rebirthing breathwork, positive thinking, immersing myself in books I loved and attending a Women Who Love Too Much support group, I was able to both quit the smoking and heal the co-dependency.

Let's look at the importance of feeling our feelings:

- Feeling your feelings can heal you.

- Feeling your feelings enables you to step out of any addiction.

- Feeling your feelings means being in touch with yourself.

- Feeling your feelings means your emotional energy is moving and healthy.

- Feeling your feelings means you do not suppress how you feel.

- Feeling your feelings means you do not 'dump' your emotions on others through yelling, shouting or making them cry.

- Feeling your feelings points to what thoughts you are thinking, making you aware of whether or not they are serving you well.

Do you know what feelings cause you to binge? For one person it might be anger and stress. For another it could be fear and boredom. I often say that eating when full is our means of coping with a life with which we are not fully satisfied, and as we stop when full, thus feeling our feelings more intensely, our feelings too, may be telling us just that – that we are living a life with which we are not fully satisfied. So, our task here is to change our perspective on our life whilst working towards altering and changing those aspects of our life that we can alter and change, even in small ways. Taking even tiny steps towards altering and changing one aspect of your life can be tremendously fun, healing and exciting, revitalizing and can renew you in the shifting winds of positive, self-inspired evolution.

Feelings are there to be felt, challenges are there to be resolved. Our constant goal is to feel feelings and resolve challenges, not live a life devoid of feelings and challenges. Although a problem-free life may seem tempting at times, there are no riches in a life devoid of feelings and challenge. There is no growth or expansion in a life devoid of feelings and challenge. Strength, wisdom, contentment, inner and outer riches all come from resolving difficult feelings and challenges. And as we master the fine art of resolving, we are also healing our weight problem.

Many people believe that self-acceptance will magically appear once they get slim. But the harsh reality is, many of us *have* become slim, only to realize, that our self-acceptance, is still at a critically low level. So, if being slim doesn't automatically make us more accepting of ourselves then what does? Well, self-acceptance is a frame of mind, and like all frames of mind is dependent on our thoughts, how we think about ourselves, positive or negative, condemning or understanding, forgiving or blaming. Therefore your mind, is the source, of your self-acceptance.

Self-acceptance is about no longer making a problem out of the self. Self-acceptance is about embracing who you are, without being blind to your faults but not beating yourself up about them either. Self-acceptance allows a general *working on our faults* in a compassionate way with the best methods we have at our disposal at any given moment in time. Self-acceptance is gentler and kinder than self-criticism, and certainly helps us move forward in life.

If you can say to yourself in a genuine, heart-felt way, as you would to a beloved child or friend, I love you – then you have cracked it. You have the secret to life, love, happiness, along with the ability to deal with anything life throws your way, good, bad and indifferent, you'll be able to handle it because you are strengthened by your genuine love for yourself. Having this genuine good feeling towards yourself is a good thing, it makes you a kinder, nicer, more loving, fair, understanding person to be around, for you cannot help but extend that love to others.

Being fabulous is not allowed. To have it all, is not allowed. This is the subtle message many of us learned as children. And even to be yourself is not allowed. We learned that we had to do as Mum, Dad or teacher tells us, and there was not much room for what we wanted to do. When we shone, maybe we were dampened down. When we expressed exuberance at a subject or activity at school that inspired us and brought us joy, maybe we were ignored, diminished or even criticized. So, as adults we have a lot of fear about being the woman that goes for her heart-felt goals and maybe even starts to - *have it all.*

If every area of your life is going well except your weight, then to have a slim body would mean – you *have it all*. This may be an unconscious, uncomfortable issue for you and if so, you can deal with it by addressing the fears around it, such as, the jealousy of others, and people not liking you. You can ask yourself – How do I deal with it when a friend or co-worker acts jealous? How do I deal with it, when someone resents my success? And, are there other ways of thinking and responding to people who act jealous, in either subtle or overt ways? The bottom line is – Do not allow the discomfort or tactics of manipulation from others be any reason for you to stay overweight or dampen down your desire to achieve the life you want.

The slim woman is a stereotype. A major subconscious urge for many of us who have suffered from, or are currently suffering from compulsive eating, *is* a struggle with the stereotypical image of the slim woman. When I was a compulsive eater, I was so obsessed with becoming a ridiculous seven and a half stone (a target weight that was actually *underweight* for my five-foot-four height) I never imagined that I might have some ambivalence about being the slim, attractive, young woman. It was not until I explored the negative and even fearful aspects of becoming the slim, attractive, woman – the stereotype – that I was able to become permanently slim (a happy eight and a half stone, and ideal for my height).

Who am I? I realized I wanted to be me and not a stereotype. I was only nineteen when I tackled my habit of *eating when full* and obsession with size, in this holistic, non-diet way; so asking myself - Who am I? - was quite interesting. A private education had, funnily enough, only left me with a basic education, not really serving me well in many respects, but it was a good enough foundation. The subliminal message from my 1980's rural, Irish, culture was that you get married, become a housewife and have children. I was pretty much okay with that, but I had a rebellious streak, and was not quite sure where this cocktail of contradictions would take me. With my first job as a humble sales assistant I was able to *meet people* and because I knew I was a *people person* this was quite a good job for me. The job also got me away from the confines of the isolated farm that was my parental home. A bit of breathing space, and room to start *finding myself* was what life was giving me, and it was perfect.

In the town where I worked, the local secondhand bookstore proved to be my salvation, for there I found the most interesting and wonderful books on feminism, spirituality, and I guess what could be described as pop-psychology. These were books written by people who definitely thought outside the box, and I loved it. In particular, the book Fat Is a Feminist Issue by Susie Orbach, had a great influence on me and started me on the road to being aware of what feelings caused me to overeat.

So reading these books gave me a string of new ideas and tools to help me along my way. My new positive identity was beginning to form. I realized I was a young woman with an interest in holistic pursuits. I was already vegetarian, and through the books I started to practice a little Yoga. I emersed myself in this new world of self-help, pop psychology and alternative health; really appreciating how the topics in these books fired my interest and were a huge, life-changing, inspiration to me. The biggest thing that helped me further answer the question – Who am I? – was, and still is, the all-important questions that I purposely, repeatedly mention throughout this little book, in an effort to convey them deeply into your way of living: *What feeling is this?* And – *Given the fact I feel this way what would I like to do now?* These questions, I ask *all* my workshop participants and one-to-one clients to ask themselves, for, not only are they quite literally the whole course condensed into eighteen words, they are a formula that is a real winner in helping you discover who you are, and free you from eating when full, and the resulting excess weight.

So spend a moment reflecting on your interests. Spend a moment asking yourself - *Who am I?* I am not a stereotype, I am not a cardboard cutout, I am me, with quirks and interests, imperfections and flaws. I love this, and I dislike that, I am an avid follower of this and a distinct disbeliever in that.

Fill in the blanks, I am _____ And you will be getting to know yourself better.

Look at your list, and for the things you would like to change:

For example: I am a little grumpy in the mornings. I am in a job I don't like. I am afraid to take that training course I fancy.

So, what I would say to you now is:

Own it, then change it.

Own it, transform it.

Own it, let go of it.

Ask yourself - *How can I alter, change, transform or let go of this?* And just like when we ask ourselves the question – *Given the fact I feel this way what would I like to do now?* – listen out for any intuitive guidance you might receive through repeated ideas that feel optimistic, joyful, or just, good-old-fashioned common sense.

Now look at your *I am* _____ list and tick off the good and positive ones, like, I am a good mother. I am loving home schooling my three kids. I am a good listener for I can sense that my friends get a lot from my listening to them when they are chatting with me. So now:

Own it, keep it.

Own it, cherish it.

Own it, you are it.

This is what we do with our positive attributes and activities; for our own appreciation of them *feeds* us in wonderful, priceless ways and we keep and expand the life we love to live.

And there is another way we can use this 'owning' attitude, with a third *I am* _____ list. A list of <u>what you would like in your life</u>. So, if you want happiness write down - 'I am happy.' And, yes you've guessed it – own it.

Own it, before you even have it.

Own it, imagine it.

Own it, feel it.

You invite it into your life by *feeling you have it, before you have it*. Remember times you felt happy, daydream a daydream that *allows* you to feel happy, and thus you bring it into your life in a very real way.

So, getting to know who you are is one hurdle, and once you start to discover your own interests and heart-felt desires, the putting-them-into-practice stage naturally expands from that knowing. Reading books on what interests you, joining a night class, and attending workshops all can be done. A change or shift in career, or even where you live, may occur, as you follow your interests and heart-felt desires. Often, unexpected pleasant doors open for us and we come to be seen as people in charge of our own destiny, this can glean support from family and friends, or it might receive an indifferent reaction, overt or covert opposition, or discouragement. At this point in time we can remember the all-important truth, we are not doing this to either gain approval or rebel, we are following our own heart-felt desires because that is simply how we are choosing to live our lives, it is a choice, one we take regardless of the reactions of others. Our slim, healthy weight, and our good physical, mental and emotional health depend on it.

Depending on your own individual upbringing, the extent to which you were allowed to be who you wanted to be, feel and express what you needed to feel and express, and do what you loved to do, to a degree determines how healthy and happy you are today. However, even with an abusive past we can heal and grow out of that pain. Eating when full often becomes a coping mechanism picked up in childhood from overeating parents, as a way of dealing with the emotional pain of dysfunctional, family dynamics. But whatever habits we've picked up can be dropped as we work on ourselves and our own personal healing.

It's called self-love and it's powerful! It is a solid foundation on which to build your life. It is the strength to value and pursue your heart-felt desires. It is the ability to be self-supporting and self-reliant. It is a constant source of forgiveness of self and others. It gives birth to the ability to alter and change anything about your own self, or life, you wish to change. It allows you to accept others as they are, and empowers you to leave others if, how they are, is abusive in any way.

Self-criticism is the opposite of self-acceptance. Self-criticism does not help you change your size and shape. Self-criticism makes you feel bad about your size and shape. Self-criticism makes you feel bad about yourself when you are doing the very best you can to deal with your weight problem. Self-criticism depletes your energy and keeps you stuck in the eating patterns you wish to change. Change is not easy at the best of times, and self-criticism makes it even harder. Notice any self-critical thoughts and notice how they make you feel.

Self-acceptance and change go hand-in-hand. Accepting where you are, without the harsh judgment of self-criticism causing you pain and shame, you alter and change more easily. In looking at self-acceptance, we are looking at the attitude and frame of mind that makes change easier.

You are in the process of changing your eating patterns. The pattern of *eating when full* is to be changed into the pattern of stopping when full. Many overweight people also have the habit of not eating when they are, in fact, physically hungry, and this needs to be changed into the pattern of eating when hungry, stopping when full. Two things help us change ingrained patterns of behavior (1) Resolve those feelings underlying the pattern and (2) A non-judgmental, self-accepting attitude towards that pattern we'd like to change.

Eat what you fancy when physically hungry. We usually go through an unhealthy food phase at the beginning of practicing eating when hungry and stopping when full, simply because I'm telling you to *also eat exactly what you want*, when you want, as long as you are physically hungry. This unhealthy food phase happens especially if you have spent years denying yourself certain foods, usually the high calorie, sweet or oily foods such as pastries, butter, chocolate, sweets or biscuits. I've even had clients that would avoid bananas and peanuts, relatively healthy foods, in my opinion, compared with sugary cakes, biscuits or bread. Do not panic if you are seriously drawn, when hungry, to eat these 'unhealthy' foods. If you keep focusing on *stopping when full* you will not gain weight, you may feel sluggish, but you will not gain weight. Let your focus be primarily on stopping when full and feeling your feelings, over and above, worrying about the *type* of foods you are eating. Once you have reassured yourself sufficiently that you will never again deny yourself *any* type of food, you will automatically start to desire the healthier foods. Oily, sweet, or calorie-laden foods will be eaten, but in an *inner-motivated moderation* born from the experiential knowledge, that to live off chips and chocolate, actually feels awful.

Loving food: People often say to me – 'My problem is I love food.' I reassure them that *loving food* is not the problem, *eating when full* is the problem. I've been naturally slim for over twenty years now and I adore food. So do not worry, you will still love food, you will simply no longer eat it when you are full.

You will simply no longer be using it as a means by which you suppress your emotions. You will move into eating when hungry and stopping when full, and loving the tastes and textures all the more because you are hungry when you eat. You will discover the wonderful truth that food does indeed, taste amazingly good, when you are hungry when you eat it.

Feeling feelings is the bottom line alternative to *eating when full* because of them. *Feeling feelings* gets you slim and keeps you slim.

Life gives us challenges to be overcome. Life brings us lessons to be learnt. We run away from our lessons, challenges and feelings when we eat when full.

Feeling our feelings, learning our lessons and facing our challenges *is* part and parcel of living a fulfilling life. Life brings up feelings to be felt. Life brings us natural permanent weight loss when we stop when full, and *stopping when full* is easier when the reason you *ate when full*, has been dealt with.

It is good to seek help in dealing with life's challenges that cause you to eat when full. Depression, boredom and stress can all be dealt with in ways other than eating when full. Find those other ways through using the methods outlined in this book and my other two books True Slimness and Guidelines for Healing Your Eating Habit. Use the amazing resource of You Tube for finding videos and audios on personal development and natural health and healing. One of my personal favorites is Hay House Radio on www.hayhouseradio.com, a free and wonderful self-help resource.

What to eat? We all know what to eat, we all know what we *should* be eating. We all know which foods are good foods and which foods are bad foods, we all know what foods are healthy for us and what foods are not healthy for us. It is the *difficulty in practicing what we know* that is the problem here. Lifestyle and eating habit changes are rarely easy unless we address the emotional reasons why we had that unhealthy habit or lifestyle to begin with.

So, again I would bring you back to our much-repeated pair of questions – What feeling is this? And - Given the fact I feel this way what would I like to do now? For the answers to these questions can help so, so much. Practice them as soon as you put this book down, memorize them and get into the new habit of asking yourself them daily, especially every time you crave food when full and you will be well on your way to natural, permanent, slimness.

Peace and permanent slimness lie in the resolving of the emotional stuff that has the potential to drive us to the fridge when full. The way to a fulfilling life is opened when we stop when full and involve ourselves in activities, books, friendships, studies, work and pastimes we are interested in.

Remind yourself often - *Eating when full* serves a purpose – it suppresses feelings we do not want to feel. Feeling, and dealing with feelings is the antidote.

Life has a way of fulfilling itself – Ask yourself today – What would a fulfilling life look like to me?

Make a list of what activities would fulfill you. Pick one. What is one, small, step, towards incorporating that activity into your life? And simply take it.

Eating when full is self-defeating behaviour. It defeats us in our task of losing excess weight for good. It defeats us in achieving and maintaining good health to a greater or lesser extent. It defeats us in being able to resolve our feelings, for it merely suppresses them, leaving them festering below our level of awareness in the very fat cells of our bodies. Unresolved emotional issues, suppressed feelings, unmet challenges and unmet needs *are* the root cause of all ill health and addiction in my opinion.

We indulge in self-defeating patterns of behaviour like eating when full which causes excess weight, because there is a pay off. This pay-off is often hidden. We are not consciously aware that our *eating when full* will serve to – for example - protect us – but if we have a subconscious association between fat and protection, then that idea of *fat providing protection* will be there, every time we feel threatened, and will produce the urge to overeat. So we must look at how we *deal* with this issue of our own *protection and safety*. Ponder the concept by asking yourself - How do I ensure I am safe?

There is nothing else to do, so we indulge in the addiction. Coming out of addiction is all about creating *something else to do* that you enjoy - and doing that! Also, of course, as I have mentioned before, but it bears repeating due to its phenomenal importance, *resolving* any emotional issue that the addiction may have been enabling you to suppress. So again, key components here, in dismantling any addiction and specifically *eating when full*, is *create and resolve*. Create involvement in what you are interested in, and resolve uncomfortable emotions.

Drum and dance I believe are crucial parts of society. To drum and dance with others has a bonding effect, and a cleansing-negative-emotions effect. It can also be an expression of positive emotions. It is a way of getting and allowing your spirit into your physical body *and* it keeps you physically fit. It is no coincidence that there is an upsurge in classes on Nia Dance, Tango, and Zumba, as well as wonderfully fun drumming and percussion workshops. Natural voice choirs are also an extension of this *joining together* in a form of creative expression of harmony. Think of it, when you drum with a group of people your whole focus is on *being in rhythm with one another* so the overall sound is good. Take that lesson into life – our focus is on being in rhythm, in harmony with one another as we each live and involve ourselves in our own individual realms of interest, thus simultaneously expressing who we are, as individuals, and as a unified entity.

Often there is a tendency to *swap addictions* along the journey of recovery from the compulsion to eat when full. That means, instead of eating when full, we start to drink a little extra wine, or smoke more if we are already smokers. Or if we have given up smoking, the urge to smoke again may return with intensity. Smoking won't help, to drink alcohol won't help – you may lose weight but start (or increase) those other bad habits. Being slim with an increased drinking or smoking habit, is really not the answer, and, in my opinion not success. So if you find yourself drawn to indulge in *any other addiction,* or feel you are still distracting yourself from your emotional issues and feelings, simply face your feelings by asking our old, reliable, addiction busting questions - What feeling is this? And – Given the fact I feel this way what would I like to do now? The healthy answers to these questions will put you firmly back on the right track.

Habits of distraction are what I would call minor addictions and what we are to be aware of as we give up eating when full and start to lose the excess weight for good. For we are now firmly on the road of gaining practice at feeling our feelings more intensely, while tackling both the major problems and minor hiccups of life in new, exciting and creative ways.

Examples of habits of distraction: Flicking through a magazine, or flicking through TV channels full of things you are not really interested in. Playing video games, incessantly talking, gossiping etc. From the minor buzz from a mug of strong coffee or cocoa, to the sugar high of too much cake, all these are *habits of distraction* that we can become aware of, as we fine-tune our awareness of ourselves, our actions, and the effect they have on our bodies and our lives. But this is advanced level stuff, and generally simply unfolds for the individual as she continues her journey of freedom from *food when full,* and any other addiction, she may be drawn towards.

If you are a person that says 'Well I don't have any other problems except my weight.' Or 'My life is going really well, it is *just my weight* that is the problem,' then it is a shock when you start to cut back on the food you eat (in an effort to lose weight) and find that you feel a little off, or uncomfortable, or suddenly more aware of some half-buried issue between you and your husband, co-worker, boss or mother-in-law for example. You are faced with the previously hidden fact that certain aspects of your life are not as perfect as you thought. You have problems. This can be hard to wrap your brain around, and you may feel resistant to this uncomfortable awareness, as it highlights new difficulties to be dealt with. As I mentioned before, but it bears repeating – Knowing, in advance, *that emotional resolving is part and parcel of the journey to permanent slimness*, is important preparation for handling those emotions when they come up. This knowing, tends to ease the *tendency to swap addictions in an effort to deal with that emotional stuff* that life does indeed throw our way, and encourages us to look at healthy alternative ways of dealing with that self-same emotional stuff.

Co-dependency is basically obsessing about how our partner should change rather than looking at ourselves. Our relationship may turn sour and we refuse to leave, or we realize that it should have ended two years ago but still we refuse to leave – this is being co-dependant. Staying with a partner who is either physically, emotionally, sexually or psychologically abusive - *is* co-dependency. He is the object of our addiction just as much as *food when full,* drugs, alcohol or cigarettes. And it is all about avoiding our own emotional stuff. Living a life full of drama as the norm, can also, serve as a huge distraction from our own emotional issues and the often daunting, sometimes even painful task of resolving them. But it is more painful to stay stuck in the cycles of addiction and the lifestyle that that involves.

So again, I will mention this truth - Addiction serves a purpose, it helps us deal with our unresolved feelings, issues and emotional stuff, but in an unhealthy, self-abusive way. To give up addiction successfully, we have to find another way to serve that purpose of dealing with our feelings, issues and emotional stuff – a healthier, self-nurturing way.

Morning musing. Today a lovely silence again prevails, permeating everything like a new dawn, a new birth, all is still – the pure primordial feeling of stillness to be found in those close to nature and in the drug-free, birthing mother, for a drugged birthing mother takes on the drug, not the stillness of birth, or maybe that is something that cannot be suppressed only hidden for one lifetime. In the next lifetime maybe the mother can experience a drug free, pain free birth, for life gives us infinite chances to be who we need to be, who we want to be, and to experience what we do not think is possible now, but later, take on as ordinary and nice to experience.

I am at peace now within my soul in this quietness of the morning air damp with rain. I think of the mother horse and her foal that happily sniffed at my face and nose yesterday, they were lovely, so aware of life, so peaceful, friendly and curious. I love horses, beautiful creatures they are, as all animals are, wonderful, unconditional love they have. When kept in their natural state, in a herd, horses show us their great loyalty to the herd, they embody beauty, power, passion, freedom and most important the protection of the young. They are energy healers too. They can, with their noses, hone in on where the energy is blocked on another horse or human being, and will endeavour to shift that energy through breathing on that area, grooming or even giving you a little push. Being with horses is what I love and have the opportunity to experience thank goodness. It helps keep me addiction-free, and slim.

Natural childbirth has also been an interest of mine. In the months and even years before and after I gave birth I spent time reading about it, as well as experiencing it myself.

So, what do you love, and have the opportunity to do? It will be part of what keeps you addiction free, and slim.

Leave some food on your plate if you are a person who simply has to finish off every bit of food on their plate regardless of hunger or fullness. Allow your fullness sensation to be the <u>sole authority</u> as to when you stop eating. And that fullness sensation, could kick in three-quarters way through a meal. That fullness sensation, could kick in half way through your main course at a fancy restaurant, where the food is very expensive, and extremely delicious. Awkward isn't it? To stop at that point. Inconvenient to say the least. Anyway, this is our difficult task, as we give up eating when full. Will that food go to waste if you do not eat it? No, not if they give you a doggie bag. Will you have wasted your money? Only if you consider shoving food into your already full stomach a good idea, and I think we have already realized that it tends to make us overweight and bloated. I don't think it is a waste of money to <u>not</u> be overweight or bloated, and bring home a doggie bag. This is the price we pay to be slim, to change a habit, to be in good health with good digestion, treating the body with kindness. And you will enjoy that doggie bag food later when genuinely physically hungry.

Emotions rule our world in so many ways. The books of Ester and Jerry Hicks state that our emotions set a vibration within our very being, and that vibration attracts unto itself that which is like unto itself. Suppressed emotion is a heavy vibration that literally makes us physically heavy when we eat when full because of those emotions rather than processing them in healthy ways. The books, You Tube Videos and DVDs of Ester and Jerry Hicks are a valuable resource in learning how to handle emotions in healthy ways and in mastering them create a life you desire.

Look back on the last time you had a binge. Ask yourself – What emotion would I have felt, if I had stopped when full? That is what you are dealing with – that emotion! The way forward is learning how to handle that emotion, learning how to *feel* that emotion, learning how to change the negative, dull, pessimistic thoughts that are associated with that emotion, with the help of the books or You Tube videos of Louise Hay, Dr Wayne Dyer, or Byron Katie. Thus you gain added resources to help you cease eating when full because of that emotion.

Creativity and living the life you love, being involved in activities you love, getting paid for activities you love, this is possible for each and every one of us. And the journey towards that, is intimately connected with being free from eating when full, excess weight and any addiction.

As I mentioned before - two things can be said to *heal* addiction, they are - creativity and resolving. They can also be said to be the *hallmark* of an addiction-free life. So creativity and resolving are both the *journey and the destination*.

An addict does not resolve her emotional issues, she suppresses them to a greater or lesser extent. She is not living a life she loves, she is not creative in a really grounded healthy way because all the unresolved emotional stuff gets in the way.

Ask yourself - What am I interested in? What do I love? What books, if any, do I love to read? Take yourself off to the library for a few hours or an afternoon even, especially if it has a study area, and just browse, choose a book or two, dip in, and read the first few pages. Do you find it interesting? If you don't, then put it down, leave it back on the shelf, and choose another.

Looking on the Internet for local night classes and browsing through your options is a great way to involve yourself in what you might be interested in. Notice if any one course takes your fancy. Sign up and do not worry if you want to drop out half way through, I have dropped out of many classes before I discovered what I was truly interested in, but the short time that I did spend at each individual class nevertheless gave me something valuable that I found useful later on in my life. And from all of them, the people I met were a tremendous blessing, for meeting people always gives you something. We learn about ourselves through our interactions with others.

When you involve yourself in doing what you love you can ask for help, and those interested in the same pursuits will help you. It is natural, and rational, that people interested in the same things will gravitate towards one another. Clubs, Internet forums and chat rooms exist solely due to this. We all know how great it is to talk with someone who is 'on the same wavelength' and our lives are truly enhanced by regular meetings with like-minded friends. We feel understood, supported and our ideas cherished. This is fertile ground for the flourishing of that particular interest and meaningful interactions with others.

The winds of change are certainly blowing around me today! Living up on a small hillside in Wales I am no stranger to whistling winds in winter. Today they are blowing musically in lovely gusts and crescendos like a symphony of movement in the air. So I've opened my windows and doors to allow the gusts to freshen the whole house. In such an atmosphere the thought 'Winds of Change' keeps springing to mind.

The time is ripe for change and shift – the outer is simply reflecting the inner. As I've been using various tools to move my life forward in the direction I desire to go (tools, which I mentioned here, in my other books and teach in my workshops and one to one consultations) I feel I'm navigating the waters of the unknown. This is not new, I've experienced this many times as change has been a big part of my life. The first major change having been my recovery from compulsive eating over twenty years ago. So know, that as you lose weight this way – by eating when hungry, stopping when full, and addressing the emotional issues that can cause you to eat when already full, you too, are going to feel a little like you are venturing into the unknown. Let me reassure you that it is okay, you do find your way. What is being asked of you, is to develop a greater trust in yourself and your intuition to guide you every step of the way. Step by step, you simply know what to do, and you allow yourself to make mistakes as you go for what you would like to be, do and have in your life. Everyone can have a slim body, everyone can stop when full, but it will *feel* different. To be a person who stops when full *is different* to being a person who eats when full, so allow the journey to go at its own pace. It is nothing less than an inner and outer transformation that you are going through. You will lose weight at a speed that is right for you, and it comes as a direct result of (yes you know it) eating when hungry and stopping when full and resolving those emotional issues that have the potential to drive you to the fridge when full.

I venture deep into the awareness of my beingness. I find the inner esoteric way and I find the outer peaceful, fulfilled way. You can tell I like meditation! When you meditate you can connect with an inner beingness and stillness that will enable you to live your life from a place of calm, and find your way to live your own life, no matter what is going on around you. Meditation is practically mainstream now, and a valuable life tool in my opinion, from chanting (meditation on sound) to focusing on your breath, to guided visualization, there are many classes available in your local community or nearby town. It causes you to dig deep within your own self to find peace, it helps you be in contact with and resolve emotional issues that need clearing up. It is *going within* rather than *running away from* the self. It is a very healing practice. Many years ago I had an experience of extreme lack that meditation helped me tremendously with, and out of this experience I wrote my biography. It sprang from a time in my life when I had nothing, literally nothing materially. It was a testing time that ultimately reaped great blessings and a blossoming for me and my life because it had caused me to *go deep* and do some soul serching. The experience felt like what the Buddhists call – The Void. It was like a black, depth of soil, and I was the seed in that soil, growing somehow towards the light, not knowing how, not knowing when or even where that final blossoming would take place, but one step at a time I held on to, and saw the success of my heart-felt desires – to home school my child and continue to be a writer.

With no, or very little light, sometimes just a sense of where the light might be, eventually the situation of lack shifted and changed as I continued to take action on what felt like what might be a way forward, and, over time, my life evolved into a living, breathing life that I was very, very happy with - a life with like-minded, home-schooling friends, a lovely house, writing, horses and adequate financial means.

So again, the point I am making here is that this is not the quick fix, although I wouldn't discount a rapid recovery because it does indeed sometimes happen that way. What I am trying to say is – This method is not a band aid, it is real healing. So, whatever the speed of your recovery, this still is not a *get slim quick and your life is perfect* message. What I am teaching is a way of living, and a slim way of living, an authentic way of living, a way of living that is a thousand times better than a compulsive, overweight, way of living; and I speak from experience, but you will not be spared difficulties, you are not spared the ups and downs of life. What you are spared is the inability to cope effectively and healthily with those ups and downs, and that alone, makes a world of difference. You give yourself a slim you - a slim, healthy *you*, a *you* that deals with, and looks at things slightly differently, than the compulsive, overeating, you.

Our emotions are one thing, our eating habits are another. The resolving of emotional issues and the involving oneself in that which you are interested in, is the groundwork, and the process of living a life free from overeating and any other addiction for that matter. To be aware of and resolving our emotional stuff is necessary, because it is often, the unresolved emotions of insecurity, fear, resentment, guilt or anger (to name but a few) that can prevent us from going out there and involving ourselves in what would ironically meet many of our emotional needs. The choice will always be there. Do we go back to the quick fix of watching too much TV, overeating, drinking, smoking etc. etc., etc., ad nauseam? All distractions from the pain that is preventing us from living fuller lives and meeting our emotional needs appropriately. The answer is *feel* the pain and do it anyway. A bit like a paraphrase of Susan Jeffer's classic book Feel the Fear and Do It Anyway, another

excellent resource to help you along your way,
feeling your feelings as you live your life your way –
a naturally slim way, an addiction-free way.

It doesn't matter so much what it looks like. For
example: If we feel moved to tears when watching a
film at the cinema with friends, we allow the tears to
flow. Okay, when we emerge from the cinema we
may look like we've been crying, but how we look is
secondary to the importance of allowing the emotion
to flow and be felt.

Another example: If we want to leave a conversation
half way through because we feel it is brewing into
an argument that we do not want to be involved in -
we leave. We may make a polite excuse, or simply
take a trip to the bathroom, grab our coat and leave,
seriously considering getting new 'friends.'

Our actions are no longer solely to look good, our
actions reflect *a lack of worry* about how we look,
and display a living, breathing, importance, that is to
do with how we feel. We are valuing how we feel.
We are deeming how we feel about things as

important and valid even though, previously, it may have been dismissed by parents, teachers, or spouses as unimportant.

Often when we involve ourselves in losing excess weight, it is about how we look. Losing weight *this way* is about how we *feel*. High self-acceptance ensures that we view ourselves as okay now at this moment in time. With high self-acceptance it is like we are giving ourselves the love and approval we never got from our mother or father, siblings, friends or teachers. Accepting yourself now, as you are, paves the way for you to become slim and heal the sorrow of any *lack of appropriate attention* in the past. And do not worry, we all have had some *lack of love, attention or approval* in our past, but through using affirmations we can raise our self-acceptance thus allowing a more positive sense of self, regardless of dysfunctional past experiences. Affirm daily: I accept myself.

So high self-acceptance allows us to more easily take the emotional ride of losing weight this way, unperturbed by how *it looks,* or how *we look*, we do start to act, and react, a little bit more *on our own behalf and in line with our heart-felt desires,* rather than stuffing them down and pretending everything is all right when it isn't. Rather than keeping silent, we speak up. Rather than say no when we really want to say yes, we say yes – not worrying about how it looks, just going with the feelings of what is right and true for ourselves. Thus moving into a life we no longer have to binge-eat to cope with.

Where does the pain come from? From where springs the discomfort we have with ourselves? It is too easy to blame our overweight bodies for that pain. Your body size, though it may be a source of angst, concern, and bad feeling for you, is not the *only, or true source* of uncomfortable feelings or any unease in your life. The source ultimately is from past painful experiences and our difficulty in processing them in healthy ways. There is however healing power in our thoughts, beliefs and therefore in the mind. I am sure you have heard of *positive thinking,* and this in no way dismisses or makes light of what hardships you went through, but is one of the many doorways to help you out of any painful emotions and overeating because of them. Try the books of Florence Scovel Shinn or Catherine Ponder.

Here is a fabulous starting point. This is a great affirmation to repeat to yourself if feeling disheartened – *Here is a fabulous starting point* – because it is! Because it is this perspective that indicates that you are no longer busy criticizing yourself for where you are, and you have shifted into realizing your ability to move from overweight to natural slimness. You are also recognizing the freeing and wonderful truth, that your excess weight can indeed, be, a temporary phenomenon. This positive perspective is a necessary foundation on which to build the eating structure of – I am physically hungry - I eat. I am physically full - I stop eating. Like the old saying – *Today is the first day of the rest of your life.* You can add to it – *And it is a fabulous starting point!*

Be active in pursuits you love. This is what many think they will do when they get slim - become active in the pursuits they love. I say 'Do it now!' Become aware of, and active in, the pursuits that you believe you will engage in when slim. Do not wait until you are slim to live the life you want to live. Allow yourself to feel the fear of stepping out of your comfort zone now, at the larger size, and begin to live the life you thought was only reserved for *the slim you* and other slim folk. The truth is, you can do it now, no matter what your size and shape, just allow yourself to do it now.

When, what your fat-self does and what your slim-self does, are one and the same thing, it is easier to cross the bridge from being an overweight person to being a naturally slim person, and it allows the results to be permanent. Now let me explain this further: Take a moment when you are at home, lie down in a comfortable position and visualize yourself weighing two stone more than you do at present. Visualize yourself at work, visualize yourself at home, then visualize yourself with friends at a social gathering. Take a few minutes to do this. And in each situation simply notice how you are behaving. Quiet, shy, fearful, vibrant, loving? Unhappy, depressed? Once you have a sense of 'who you are' at that heavier weight, imagine yourself at your slimmer or ideal weight, at work, at home and with friends, pay particular attention to the differences: Differences in your behavior and your feelings. You may find you are actually seeing two completely different versions of *you.* This is the bridge we must cross, and we do this by noticing, and becoming aware of what might feel a little uncomfortable about being slim. Unwanted attention is a common one, or feeling so light you could blow away, is another common fear. You may have to persist in visualizing yourself slim in these different situations to uncover what is a little uncomfortable in being slim, because, we are often, not consciously aware of *anything* negative in being slim, we are so busy presuming how fabulous it will be.

Likewise there is something positive in being the heavier weight, and a few attempts at the visualization can usually uncover it – the key, and I learned this from Susie Orbach's classic book 'Fat is a Feminist Issue,' is to reassure yourself that you *can deal with anything fearful* that comes up as you visualize yourself slim. Then after you have done the visualization, think of healthy, positive, life-affirming strategies to deal with those fearful situations or feelings.

As for *the positive feelings from being the heavier weight,* well promise yourself that you can take, those previously hidden, positive, attributes and vibes of being big, with you, as you get slimmer. My own personal positive of being bigger was an image of a large, immovable, Buddha, strong, in a loving, immovable, presence, able to withstand any blast of negativity directed towards her. So, anytime I felt insecure or intimidated around anyone, I would just think of that image, thus summoning up the great peace and immovability of the Buddha, and have that positive trait there, within me, as I shed my excess pounds. I was shedding my fat, but keeping that previously hidden, (subconscious) positive attribute of my fat.

I remember seeing an acquaintance of mine after she lost about three or four stone very quickly through dieting, and I was actually shocked. The reaction I felt in my body was actual shock. Her weight loss was short lived because she had done absolutely no emotional resolving along with the restriction of her food intake. She was high and dry, in a new body that she did not feel entirely at home in, a body that represented a whole new way of being that she hadn't fully explored, accepted or integrated. She had literally jumped into a new, and strange persona, a persona without a coping mechanism, for her coping mechanism had been to *eat when full.* Without the emotional work of discovering and integrating the hidden positive attributes of her fat, she also unconsciously shed those positive attributes. When the reality of this kicked in, on a subconscious level, the overwhelming urge to eat when full reasserted itself until she was occupying her fatter body again, her fatter-self stayed, her slim-self was short lived.

Who am I with excess weight? This is a vitally important question. Weight loss must be done in conjunction with the unearthing and resolving of emotional issues, in order for it to be real, and lasting.

Until we explore the emotional world of who we are fat, and who we are slim, we will never be able to lose excess weight for good. So think now: 'Who am I, when I see myself as a woman carrying excess weight? What way do I interact with my husband as I see myself as a woman carrying even more excess weight than I have now? How do I treat my kids, my mother or my boss as I imagine myself carrying the excess weight?

And likewise ask yourself: *Who am I without the excess weight?* And promise to start to bring in the positive aspects of being slim into your life now. If, as you imagine yourself slim, you realize you would join a pottery class – then do it now. You think you would wear more figure hugging clothes – wear them now. Figure hugging clothes *feel* the same fat or slim. Figure hugging clothes get the same reaction fat or slim – wear them now, and feel what they *feel like* and decide if that is a style of clothes you like. Do not let your size determine what clothes you wear. Your clothes are a reflection of *who you are,* not what size you are. So experiment with color, styles and textures and if money is a problem don't shun the charity shops, some very stylish women shop there!

Many of us when overweight, feel that our lives are lacking. But the truth is, that very few of us, fat or slim, are living the life we truly want, and if we accept that, and allow it to be a stepping-stone to where we want to be, then life has a chance to improve, and dealing with it, as it is, is more bearable. After all, when crossing a shallow stream, you do not get mad at a stepping-stone, you are thankful for it, in fact you can have a lot of fun on stepping-stones! You are getting where you want to go, step-by-step and your body *can* become slimmer step-by-step. So cease blaming and criticizing it, the size you are now is a stepping-stone to the size you desire to be. Cease criticizing the life you have now, it is a stepping-stone to where you want to be. Life can be lived this way, criticism-free and appreciation-filled, with this outlook change is made a whole lot easier.

True happiness does not come from being slim, it comes from emotional resolving. So spend some time every day doing your favorite emotional resolving practices to enjoy this precious gift called life, even if it so often feels like a burden rather than a precious gift. Give yourself the gift of freedom from the burden of suppressed emotion, for it is the suppressed emotions, and unresolved emotional stuff that makes life a burden, and clouds us from the realization that life is something precious to be treasured.

Permission is the key: What happens when you say to yourself - *I can't have that!* You want it all the more! Right? This is why I tell people: 'Give yourself permission to indulge in the object of your addiction. Give yourself permission to *eat when full* when you crave to do so. Then, once you have given yourself permission, ask yourself – Do I really want to overeat or am I ready to do some emotional resolving instead?' And ask yourself our much-repeated, power questions – What feeling is this? And Given the fact I feel this way, what would I like to do now? This actually heightens your chances of stopping when full. Ironically, through the permission to eat when full also comes the permission and the power to stop when full. It simply becomes a choice.

Ways of resolving:

- Breathwork.

- The Work of Byron Katie, the process that facilitates a change in perspective.

- Meditation – either chanting or focus on the breath.

- Affirmations.

- Sound Healing.

- Forgiveness Prayers of Howard Wills

- Hay House Radio – hayhouseradio.com

- The books of Ester and Jerry Hicks, Catherine Ponder, Cherie Martin, Geneen Roth, and Deborah King.

- Binnie Dansby www.binnieadansby.com

Feel your feelings. There is a saying - 'Know that by feeling it you are healing it.' And it is so true, the simple process of allowing yourself to feel angry, sad, unloved, bitter, disappointed, resentful etc., all those uncomfortable feelings, is authentic, real and healing, and it facilitates them passing. Yes! The very act of feeling feelings that are uncomfortable (feelings we normally do not even like to feel or admit that we even have) is healing. You are not stuffing them down in the effort to convince yourself that everything in your life is fine when it is not. It is a false thing to pretend that you are happy and plaster a smile on your face when you feel like throwing a tantrum over the latest thing your lover, spouse, sibling or boss just did. Allow yourself to *feel* what you are feeling, not necessarily expressing it, but simply breathing, relaxing and admitting to yourself, there and then, that that is how you feel, and not binge eating because of it, but in a quiet, private moment, before falling asleep at night or in the bathroom washing your hands, thinking: *I feel this way, what would I like to do now?* And pay attention to any inner, healthy, wise whispers, thoughts or wishes that bubble up to the surface, then see if you can get to work, in big or small ways on them, and see what happens to improve the situation that triggered those uncomfortable feelings.

People often say - It is *people letting me down* that is a cause of my overeating. This *'being let down'* has certainly been an issue in my own past even long after I healed my eating disorder and ceased eating when full because of people's reactions to me. The way I resolved it was this – I realized that I could expect good things from folk, things such as support, caring, positive attention, a listening ear, and a feeling of being genuinely liked.

'Don't expect so much,' was not the answer, but instead, to simply accept and appreciate each wonderful attribute that each friend, acquaintance or family member had, and be okay with them <u>not</u> being able to display other important attributes, knowing new friends would come into my life. And as I continued to expect and believe that people with the precious attribute of reliability could appear, and be present in my life, they did indeed show up. Each friend in my life provides something different in his or her own unique way. My appreciation of that, and my own <u>self-support</u> always lets me know that I am supported. Life now does indeed support me in wonderful ways and, if it happens, I can deal with the issue of being let down much more easily through changing my perspective and taking actions in line with my heart-felt desires rather than trying to change people. The most important thing is - I no longer binge-eat because someone does not support me in the way I feel they should support me.

In a support group we are doing just that - conjuring up support. We get so accustomed to our day-to-day living, and our day-to-day relating, that we may not even notice where it is not supporting us. Competition seems to be the norm and we forget that there is another way, a way of cooperation and support. We unconsciously feel that if we support another we are somehow taking that support away from ourselves, but in fact, the opposite is true – What we give out, comes back to us multiplied, or, what goes around, comes around. So when we enter a support group, or one of my workshops, the support is activated, and nourishing everyone in the unseen realms of emotion. People feel uplifted from the focus on *supporting each other* because we all know what it is like to binge eat, to turn to food when full, to even be unaware of when we are full, feeling out of control around food and not knowing why. And the coming together in the spirit of teaching, learning and support, to find our own individual answers, is a rewarding way to communicate, heal and live.

What creates that atmosphere of support is a few simple goldmine guidelines (1) No criticism. No one criticises themselves or another person in the group. (2) No interruptions. When one person is talking the others listen until that person is finished speaking. (3) Confidentiality. What is said in the group, stays with the group. If you wish to talk about something that occurred in the group, or a revelation you had, to your husband, wife or friend, you can keep confidentiality by saying '*A person I met* said / experienced....' this way privacy is kept. You never mention names. I encourage you to set up your own support group with a few friends or neighbors interested in weight loss. You could place an ad in a local newsagent's window or health shop notice board. You can hold the support group in a local church hall, community center, or even in your own front room, and thus give each other support as you work through this book together and share your experiences of recovery.

And in closing I will say again, what I wish for you is what I wished and realised for myself – the reality of nothing ever being a good enough reason to eat when full, and that is when true and lasting slimness occurs, through being - simply full.

For information on Sofia's Workshops, Books, and Skype Consultations Contact:

Facebook: Sofia Bothwell

Sofia2227@gmail.com

www.sofiabothwell.co.uk

❀

ACKNOWLEDGEMENTS

I'd like to acknowledge The Women's Therapy Centre, London and The Mary Ward Centre, London for the wonderful workshops that were part of my research into healing eating disorders and co-dependency. I'd like to thank all my clients, especially those who attended my first workshops at Violet Hill Studios, St. John's Wood, London.

And I would like to thank all my friends and clients who encouraged me to believe in the value of my work.

Om Shanti

Simply Full